Liquid Soap Making:

32 Amazing Organic Conditioning Shampoos, Moisturizing Hand Soaps and Herbal Shower Gels Recipes for All Skin Types

Table of content:

Introduction

Making your own soap is cheaper and healthier. When you make your own liquid soaps, you have the opportunity to slow your aging process, even if just a little. It's actually a natural component of the glycerine in your product. The skin is the largest organ measuring approximately 22 square feet and 60 percent of everything we put on our skin is quickly absorbed into the bloodstream. The chemicals used in soap are extremely dangerous and have been linked to cancer, reproductive issues, and allergies.

Dry skin seems to "attract" wrinkles. While this statement isn't proper scientific jargo, it does sum up what happens. Skin that is well hydrated, with, let's say glycerin, for example, will appear young-looking longer than skin that's dry.

Below are the dangerous additives

Many people have already made up their minds. The cost of exposure to these chemicals is far too high a price to pay. So instead of tolerating the commercially bought soaps, they're devising ways to avoid these substances. If you think they're overreacting, here is a list of seven of the most dangerous additives and what long-term exposure can potentially do to your body.

1. Parabens.

On the surface, parabens sound like a marvelous substance to add to soaps and other beauty products. Why? Basically, they're preservatives that retard the growth of bacteria, yeast and mold. So you may be wondering the reason anyone would consider them unwanted.

That's because they have what many medical professionals call "estrogen-mimicking properties." Specifically, parabens are linked to an increased risk of breast cancer, having been identified in the biopsies of many individuals who are diagnosed with this type of cancer. That's right, in many cancerous breasts, doctors can actually see and identify these substances.

You can easily find them in everything from makeup to, you guessed it, body washes.

2. Fragrances

Yes, fragrances. The deliciously succulent aromas we take our time choosing may be lulling ourselves into a false sense of serenity. When it comes to the generic term "fragrance," many times you may never really know what substances go into creating those appealing scents.

Companies love to keep the exact formula close to their chests, claiming nothing more than it's a secret formula or a "proprietary formula." They couldn't possibly reveal it. In this way no other company can swoop in and steal its scent – and sales.

That's all well and good from the business end, but where does that leave you, the consumer? What chemicals are you subjecting your body to that could be potentially dangerous and even fatal?

What is known is simple. These so-called signature fragrances have been linked to a host of problems, from merely annoying to downright dangerous including:

- Allergies
- Dermatitis
- Reproductive issues
- Respiratory distress

And, yes, they can be found in just about every commercial product from perfume, cologne moisturizers and body washes. It's difficult, if not impossible, to live your life without them if you use commercially bought soaps.

3. Artificial coloring

Take a good look at the label on the soap or shampoo you buy at your local drug store or even your local bath and body store. You may see substances called synthetic coloring, recognizing them mostly by initials.

4. Phthalates

I beg your pardon. How do you even attempt to pronounce a word like that? It's pronounced "they-lates," and without putting much effort into a search of commercial soaps, you can find this group of chemicals in literally hundreds of products. The manufacturers justify placing them in many products because phthalates are used to help increase the flexibility as well as the softness of plastics.

This group of chemicals is known to beendocrine disruptors as well as being associated with an increased risk in the development of breast cancer. These substances are also known to signal early breast development in young girls as well as reproductive problems in both men and women.

Since it's added fragrances, it's not necessarily printed on the labels. You'll recall the earlier group of substances aren't revealed because they're used in those "secret proprietary formulas." The scary aspect to this, then, is that you may be using it right now without even knowing it.

The fact of the matter is that phthalates can also be found in any health and beauty product from deodorants to moisturizers.

5. Sodium lauryl sulfate (SLS) and Sodium laureth sulfate

These are two separate names that you may find on your liquid soaps at home. In fact, I can practically guarantee you that if you pick up any of your personal care products that you're using right now, you'll find one or the other of these on the label. How can I be so confident?

Because they're found in more than 90 percent of beauty products and cosmetics. Think of it: 90 percent!

Sometimes simply referred to by their initials, SLS, they're known to irritate not only the skin but eyes as well. They're also well-known lung irritants.

While alone they can cause irritation, when combined with other synthetic chemicals, they potentially can interact with other chemicals to form nitrosamines – a known carcinogen.

Aside from being substances notorious for raising your risk of cancer, carcinogens, in turn, may then prompt a myriad of other issues, including damage to your kidneys and respiratory system.

Yes, they very well may be in the commercial body wash in your shower right now. And probably your shampoo, your mascara . . . and oh yes, even your child's acne-reducing products.

6. Formaldehyde

What would you say if I told you that the store-bought body wash you just brought home from your local store probably contains formaldehyde? Not only that, but it probably also has something called formaldehyde-releasing preservatives (FRPs).

As horrible and bizarre as that may seem, it's true. These particular substances aren't difficult to discover in body washes as well as a host of shampoos, conditioners, eye shadows and nail polishes.

The International Agency for Research on Carcinogens (IARC) linked this chemical to occupational related cancers, most specifically nasal and nasopharyngeal.

Formaldehyde also acts as a skin allergen and may also be detrimental to the immune system. Yes, it's almost a certainty that this substance is sitting in a bottle of body wash in your bathroom right now. If you dig just a little deeper, you'll probably find them in shampoos as well as conditioners, nail polishes, eye shadow and various cleansers.

Chapter 1. Moisturizing Hand Soaps

Calming Liquid Soap

Calming soap will keep the kids at bay when they start to get all crazy. Make them wash their hands with this stuff and they will want to settle down.

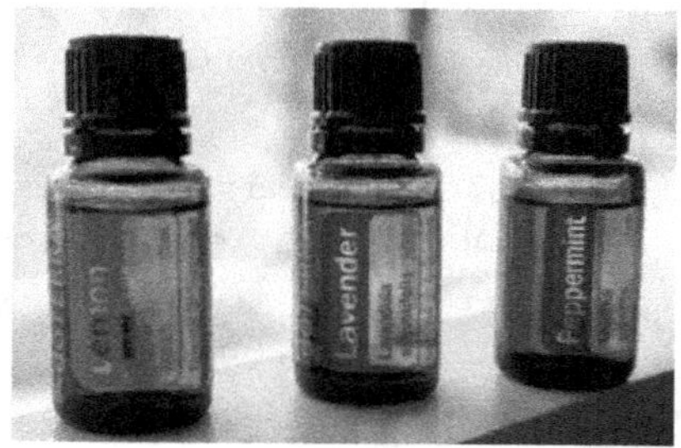

Makes: 4 12 oz. bottles

Prep: 20 minutes

Ingredients:

- Unscented grated bar of soap
- 10 cups of water
- 2 tablespoons of coconut oil
- 3 drops of lavender essential oil
- 2 drops of ylang ylang essential oil
- 1 drop of vetiver essential oil

Instructions:

1. In a large sauce pan, pour the water over the grated soap.

2. Melt.

3. Add the coconut oil.

4. Mix well.

5. Take off the stove add the fragrance oils.

6. Let cool overnight.

7. Whisk in the morning.

8. Pour into bottles.

9. Use!

Blueberry Cheesecake Liquid Soap

The scent of this Blueberry soap may make you hungry. It smells just like the sweet tasting berry and will leave your hands silky soft after you wash your hands.

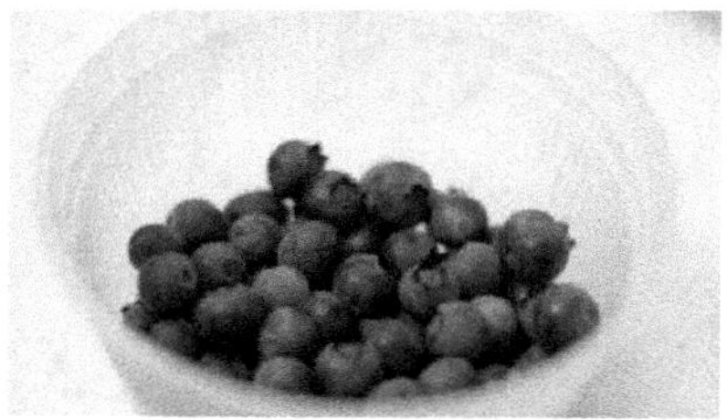

Makes: 4 12 oz. bottles

Prep: 20 minutes

Ingredients:

- Unscented grated bar of soap
- 10 cups of water
- 2 tablespoons of coconut oil
- 4 drops of blueberry fragrance oil
- 2 drops of vanilla essential oil

Instructions:

1. Place the grated soap into a large sauce pan, then pour the water over top.

2. Melt, stirring frequently.

3. Add the coconut oil.

4. Mix well.

5. Take off the stove add the fragrance oils.

6. Let cool overnight.

7. Whisk in the morning.

8. Pour into bottles.

9. Use!

Salted Caramel Liquid Soap

This soap has a salty yet very sweet smell. It will leave your hands super soft and smelling delicious.

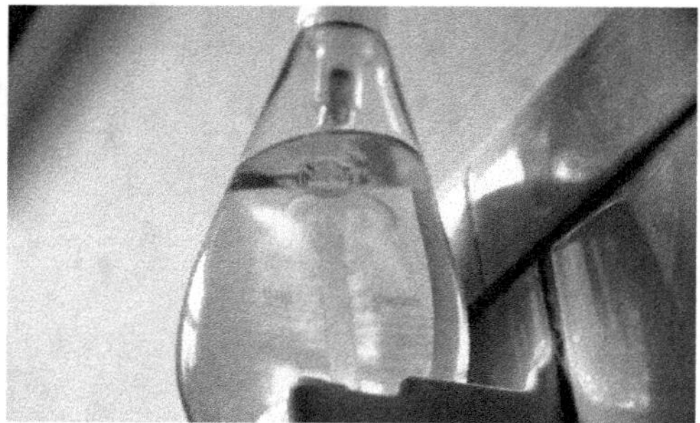

Makes: 8 oz. jar
Prep: 7 minutes

Ingredients:

- sweet almond oil
- 1 tablespoon of vitamin E oil
- distilled water
- castile soap
- Caramel fragrance oil
- sea salt fragrance oil

Instructions:

1. In an 8-ounce jar.

2. Add the distilled water first.

3. Then add the castile soap.

4. Lastly, add all the oils.

5. Shake before using.

For the Man Liquid Soap

This is the soap for the man who doesn't like the typical fruity or flowery scents. This soap smells woodsy for sure. It has great healing properties, making it perfect for those with very dry hands.

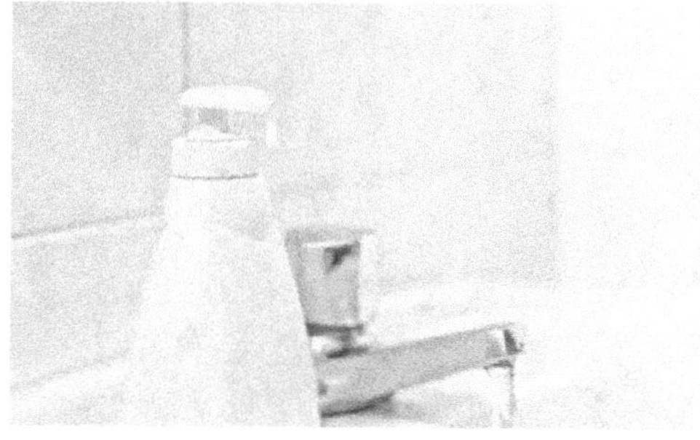

Makes: 9-pint sized jars
Prep: 20 minutes

Ingredients:

- 8 1 oz. bars of grated soap
- 2 tablespoons of vegetable glycerin
- 1 gallon of distilled water
- 1 drop fir needle essential oil
- 3 drops of allspice essential oil
- 2 drops of cedarwood essential oil

Instructions:

1. Pour water into a large pot and warm on the stove.

2. Once its heated pour in the grated soap.

3. Mix until the soap is dissolved.

4. Pour in the glycerin.

5. Add in the essential oils.

6. Transfer to a large container.

7. Let it sit overnight.

8. Whisk the next morning.

9. Start using.

Raspberry Liquid Soap

This liquid soap is great for gifts for your family and friends. It smells just like a raspberry with a hint of vanilla. It is great for any occasion.

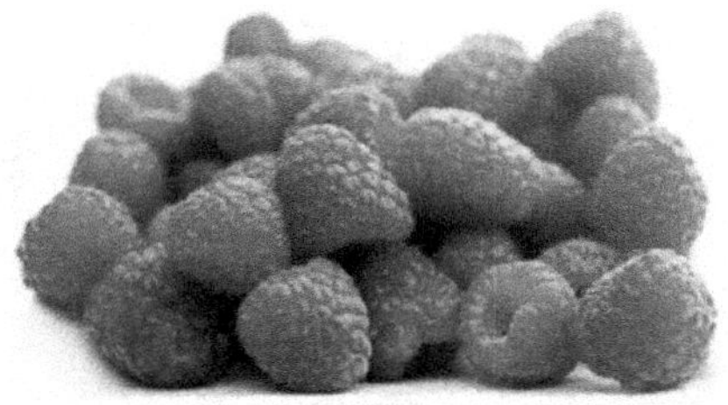

Makes: 16 ounces
Prep: 5 minutes

Ingredients:

- 1 cup peppermint castile soap
- 1 cup organic vegetable glycerin
- 2 tablespoons of castor oil
- 4 drops of raspberry essential oil
- 1 drop of vanilla essential oil

Instructions:

1. In a large bowl.

2. Mix the castile soap and the glycerin.

3. Next add all the oils.

4. Pour in a container.

5. Shake before each use.

6. Enjoy!

Trick or Treat Liquid Soap

A great decoration for Halloween as well as the smell of sweet candy. It is a combination of sweet and spicy ingredients. You will love the way it makes your skin feels after you have used it for whatever purpose you desire.

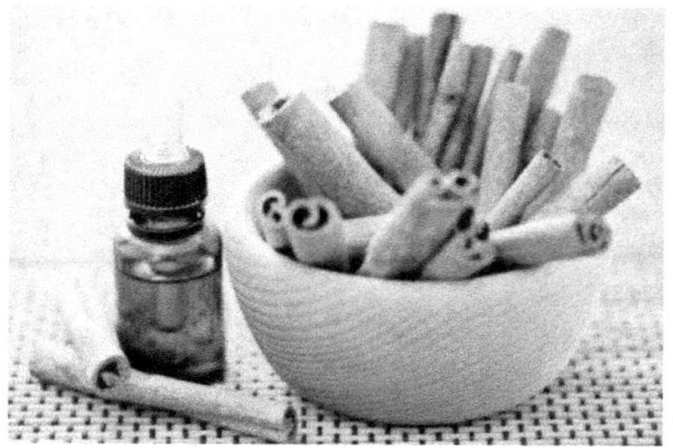

Makes: 4 12 oz. bottles
Prep: 20 minutes

Ingredients:

- Unscented grated bar of soap
- 10 cups of water
- 2 tablespoons of coconut oil
- 4 drops of cherry fragrance oil
- 2 drops of clove essential oil
- 1 drop of cinnamon essential oil

Instructions:

1. In a large sauce pan, pour the water over the grated soap.

2. Melt.

3. Add the coconut oil.

4. Mix well.

5. Take off the stove add the fragrance oils.

6. Let cool over night.

7. Whisk in the morning.

8. Pour into bottles.

9. Use!

Pink Haze Liquid Soap

Pink Haze is for the girly, girl in you! It smells so fruity and fresh. Great for a hand soap or even laundry detergent. It will smell great no matter what.

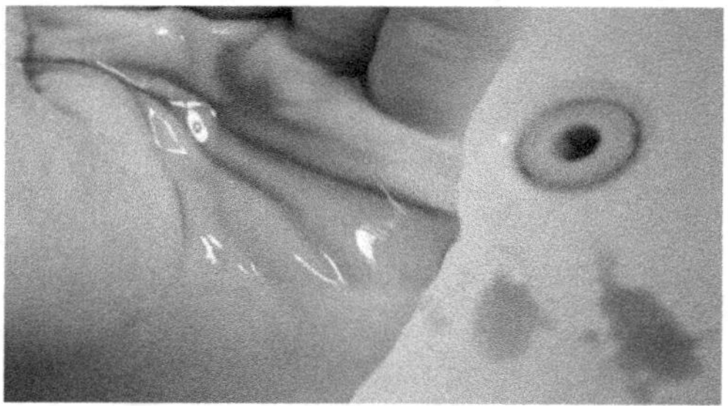

Makes: 4 12 oz. bottles
Prep: 20 minutes

Ingredients:

- Unscented grated bar of soap
- 10 cups of water
- 2 tablespoons of coconut oil
- 2 drops of blueberry fragrance oil
- 2 drops of raspberry essential oil
- 1 drop of strawberry fragrance oil
- 2 drops of vanilla extract

Instructions:

1. In a large sauce pan, pour the water over the grated soap.

2. Melt.

3. Add the coconut oil.

4. Mix well.

5. Take off the stove add the fragrance oils.

6. Let cool over night.

7. Whisk in the morning.

8. Pour into bottles.

9. Use!

Citrus Rosemary Liquid Soap

This is a great scent for any occasion! It has a clean refreshing citrus scent. It can be used for dishes or for a regular hand soap which ever you desire.

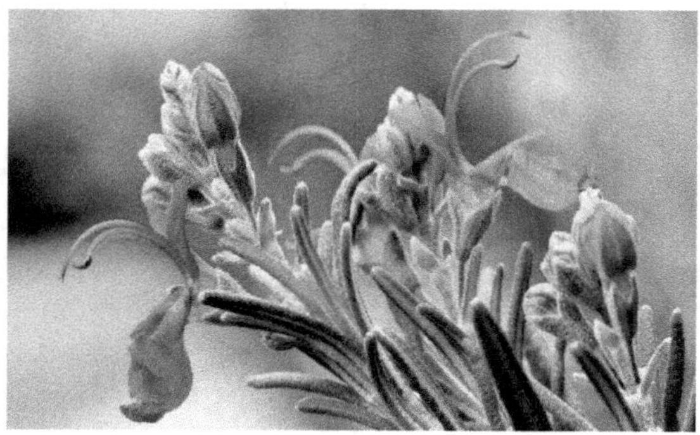

Makes: 16 ounces
Prep: 5 minutes

Ingredients:

- 1 cup unscented castile soap
- 1 cup organic vegetable glycerin
- 2 tablespoons of sweet almond oil
- 2 drops of wild orange essential oil
- 1 drop of lemon essential oil
- 1 drops of rosemary essential oil

Instructions:

1. Take a large bowl.

2. Mix the castile soap and the glycerin.

3. Next add all the oils.

4. Pour in a container.

5. Shake before each use.

6. Enjoy!

Energy Liquid Soap

Need a soap that gives you some energy? Something to give you a pick up to make it through the rest of the day. Not only does it have a great aroma it will just put you in a better mood.

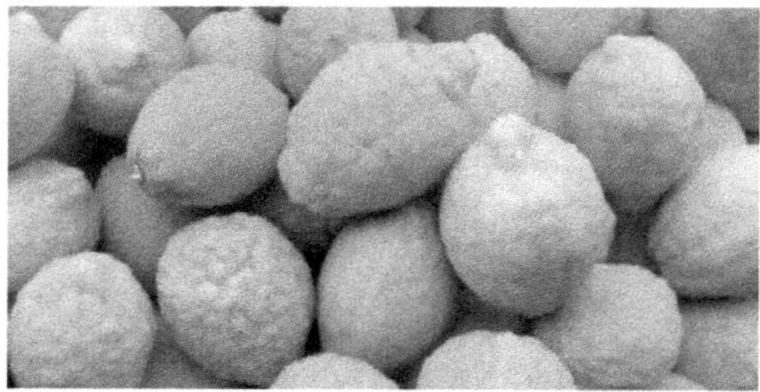

Makes: 8 oz. jar
Prep: 7 minutes

Ingredients:

- 1 tablespoon of fractionated coconut oil
- 1 tablespoon of vitamin E oil
- ½ cup of distilled water
- ½ cup unscented castile soap
- 2 drops of bergamot essential oil
- 1 drop of lemon essential oil
- 1 drop of sage essential oil

Instructions:

1. In an 8-ounce jar.

2. Add the distilled water first.

3. Then add the castile soap.

4. Lastly, add all the oils.

5. Shake before using.

Twinkle Twinkle Liquid Soap

This soap is like a good night soap. It will relax and help wind you down from a long stressful day.

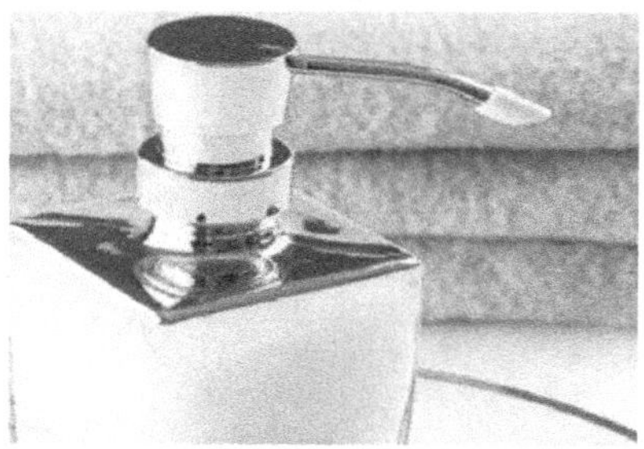

Makes: 4 12 oz. bottles
Prep: 20 minutes

Ingredients:

- Unscented grated bar of soap
- 10 cups of water
- 2 tablespoons of coconut oil
- 1 drop ylang ylang essential oil
- 4 drops lavender essential oil
- 2 drops of cedarwood essential oil

Instructions:

1. In a large sauce pan, pour the water over the grated soap.

2. Melt.

3. Add the coconut oil.

4. Mix well.

5. take off the stove add the fragrance oils.

6. let cool over night.

7. whisk in the morning.

8. pour into bottles.

9. Enjoy!!

Camu Camu Liquid Soap

If you wish you could go to the beach but can't afford to go or don't have time, then use this soap. Get swept away by the waves of the scent of this liquid soap.

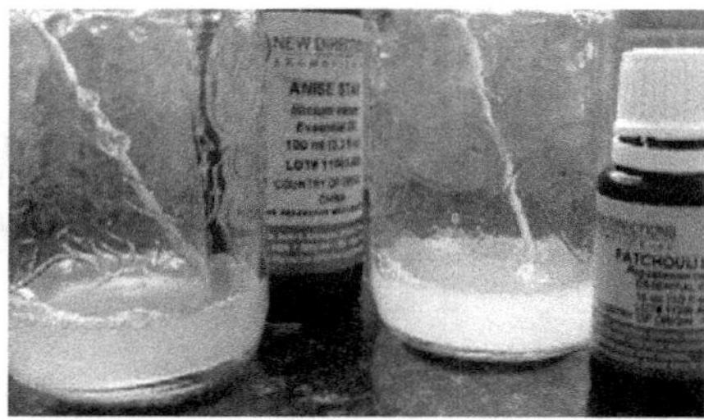

Makes: 16 ounces
Prep: 5 minutes

Ingredients:

- 1 cup peppermint castile soap
- 1 cup organic vegetable glycerin
- 2 tablespoons of grapeseed oil
- 4 drops of mandarin fragrance oil
- 3 drops of passion fruit fragrance oil
- ½ teaspoon of vanilla extract

Instructions:

1. In a large bowl.

2. Mix the castile soap and the glycerin.

3. Next add all the oils.

4. Pour in a container.

5. Shake before each use.

6. Enjoy!

Granny's Cookies Liquid Soap

Do you remember being at your grandma's house while she was baking in the kitchen? That smell of freshly baked goods forever ingrained in your mind? That familiar, comforting smell has been is exactly what this soap smell like. You can use it and remember all the fond memories you had as a child.

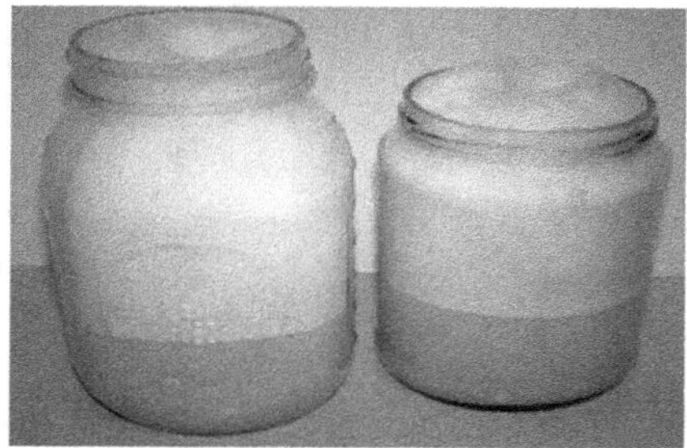

Makes: 4 12 oz. bottles
Prep: 20 minutes

Ingredients:

- Unscented grated bar of soap
- 10 cups of water
- 2 tablespoons of coconut oil
- 5 drops of sugar cookie fragrance oil
- 1 drop of tangerine essential oil
- 2 drops of vanilla extract

Instructions:

1. In a large sauce pan, pour the water over the grated soap.

2. Melt.

3. Add the coconut oil.

4. Mix well.

5. Take off the stove add the fragrance oils.

6. Let cool over night.

7. Whisk in the morning.

8. Pour into bottles.

9. Use!

Purple Potion Liquid Soap

Fruit scented anything is just so refreshing, add a hint of flowers and it's even better. This soap is awesome for anything you feel the need to use it for.

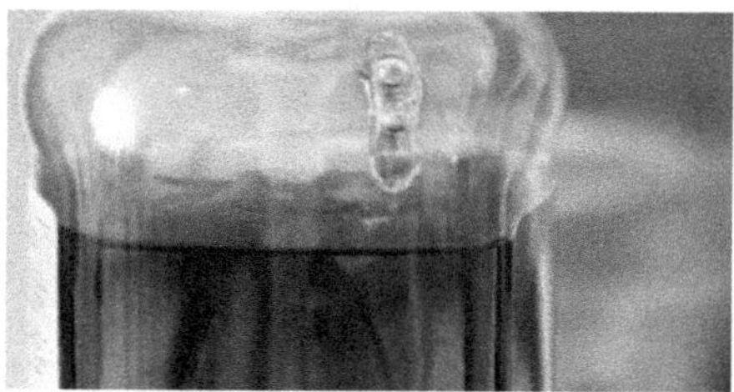

Makes: 9-pint sized jars
Prep: 20 minutes

Ingredients:

- 8 1 oz. bars of grated soap
- 2 tablespoons of vegetable glycerin
- 1 gallon of distilled water
- 3 drops of blackberry fragrance oil
- 2 drops of peach fragrance oil
- 1 drop of gardenia fragrance oil

Instructions:

1. Pour water into a large pot and warm on the stove.

2. Once its heated pour in the grated soap.

3. Mix until the soap is dissolved.

4. Pour in the glycerin.

5. Add in the essential oils.

6. Transfer to a large container.

7. Let it sit overnight.

8. Whisk the next morning.

9. Start using.

Love at First Bite Liquid Soap

This soap is like the bobbing for apples game you used to play at Halloween parties. It has a super sweet smell and the name is fun too. A great gift to give at your Halloween party.

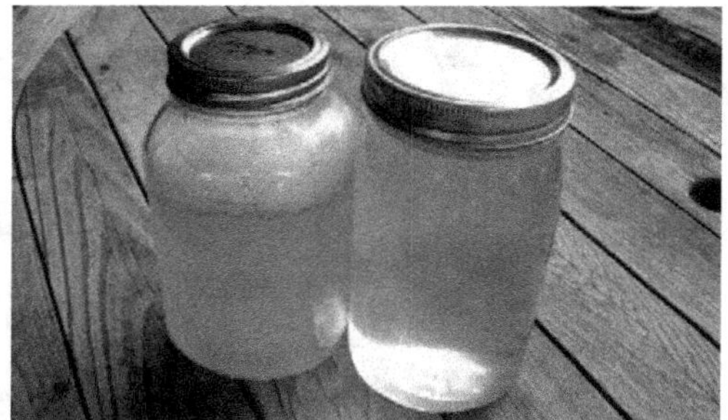

Makes: 8 oz. jar
Prep: 7 minutes

Ingredients:

- 1 tablespoon of avocado oil
- 1 tablespoon of vitamin E oil
- ½ cup of distilled water
- ½ cup unscented castile soap
- 2 drops of apple fragrance oil
- 2 drops of cherry fragrance oil
- 1 drop of vanilla essential oil

Instructions:

1. Take an 8-ounce jar.

2. Add the distilled water first.

3. Then add the castile soap.

4. Lastly, add all the oils.

5. Shake before using.

Cozy Fireside Liquid Soap

Feel like curling up next to a fire, but you don't have one? With this soap, you can close your eyes and imagine yourself curled up by a cozy fireplace. With the festive warm spice smell and the zesty ginger and cinnamon will make it seem so much more real.

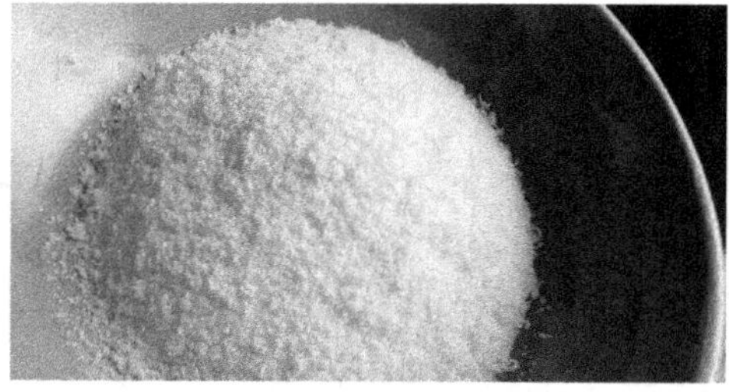

Makes: 16 ounces
Prep: 5 minutes

Ingredients:

- 1 cup unscented castile soap
- 1 cup organic vegetable glycerin
- 2 tablespoons of sweet almond oil
- 2 drops of ginger essential oil
- 2 drops of cinnamon leaf essential oil
- 1 drop of clove essential oil

Instructions:

1. In a large bowl.

2. Mix the castile soap and the glycerin.

3. Next add all the oils.

4. Pour in a container.

5. Shake before each use.

6. Enjoy!

Chapter 2. Shower Gels

Homemade moisturizing bath gels are an incredible treat for your skin. So many of the bath gels you purchase are filled with ingredients you can't pronounce, are unnecessary – and in some cases, are actually bad for your skin. You can avoid all of that by making your own shower gels.

It has been said that making your own shower gels can be difficult. I think this is all a matter of perspective. If you are looking to replicate exactly the texture of manufactured shower gels, then yes, you are going to have your work cut out for you. However, you can create a cleanser that is emollient and thick with just a few ingredients and a very simple technique. Some of the shower gels shown here will have a somewhat milky color and consistency.

This is natural and to be expected. One important thing to keep in mind is that when you make shower gels, you are adding water into the formula. Any time water is added, there is a potential for bacterial contamination. That is why antibacterial essential oils have been added to the formulas if they didn't already contain antiseptic ingredients. The amounts of these oils added is small and should not significantly affect the end result in terms of scent. You are always free to explore with other antibacterial essential oils as substitutions.

*Note: If you prefer the texture and sudsing capability of store bought shower gels, you can buy unscented shower gel bases from cosmetic supply companies and some natural food or craft stores. Just add extra moisturizing oils and scents.

Unscented Moisturizing Shower Gel

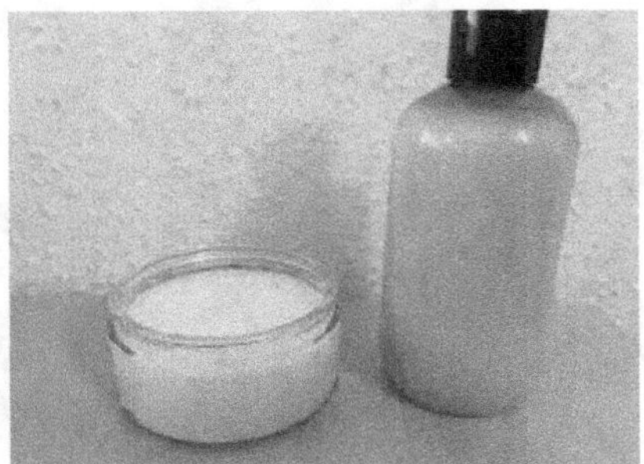

Ingredients:

- ¼ cup shea butter, melted
- ¼ cup avocado oil
- 2 teaspoons vitamin E oil
- 3 tablespoons vegetable glycerin
- 1 tablespoon xanthan gum
- 1 cup liquid castile soap
- 1 cup warm, distilled water
- Container (clean and sterilized)
- Immersion blender (or a whisk)

Instructions:

1. In a bowl, combine the melted shea butter, avocado oil, vitamin E oil, vegetable glycerin and xanthan gum. Stir gently and let the mixture sit for 5 minutes.

2. Using an immersion blender, blend the mixture until it begins to emulsify. (If you do not have an immersion blender, you can use a whisk.)

3. Add the castile soap and warm water. Whisk or quickly blend the ingredients for just a few seconds. Do not over mix and create suds.

4. Let the mixture settle for 1-2 minutes.

5. Pour the gel into an appropriate container, and store it in a cool, dry place.

6. For best results, make small batches that will be used within 14 days.

To Use:

1. Shake the container gently before use.

2. Apply the cleanser to a sponge or washcloth and cleanse the body.

3. Rinse with comfortably warm water and gently pat dry when finished.

Delicate Orange Blossom Milky Gel

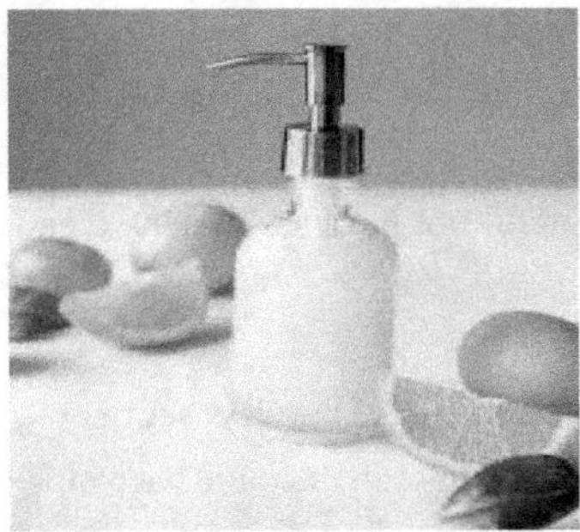

Ingredients:

- ¼ cup shea butter, melted
- ¼ cup sweet almond oil
- ¼ cup powdered milk
- 3 tablespoons vegetable glycerin
- 1 tablespoon xanthan gum
- 1 cup liquid castile soap
- 1 cup warm, distilled water
- ¼ cup orange blossom water
- 10 drops neroli essential oil
- 5 drops grapefruit essential oil (as a preservative) Container (clean and sterilized)
- Immersion blender (or a whisk)

Instructions:

1. In a bowl, combine the melted shea butter, sweet almond oil, powdered milk, vegetable glycerin, and xanthan gum. Stir gently and let the mixture sit for 5 minutes.

2. Using an immersion blender (or a whisk if you do not have a blender), blend the mixture until it begins to emulsify.

3. Add the castile soap, warm water, orange blossom water, neroli essential oil, and grapefruit essential oil. Whisk or quickly blend the ingredients for just a couple of seconds. Do not over mix and create suds.

4. Let the mixture settle for 1-2 minutes.

5. Pour the gel into an appropriate container, and store it in a cool, dry place.

6. For best results, make small batches that will be used within 14 days.

To Use:

1. Shake the container gently before use.

2. Apply the cleanser to a sponge or washcloth and cleanse the body.

3. Rinse with comfortably warm water and gently pat dry when finished.

Lavender Cocoa Butter Cleanser

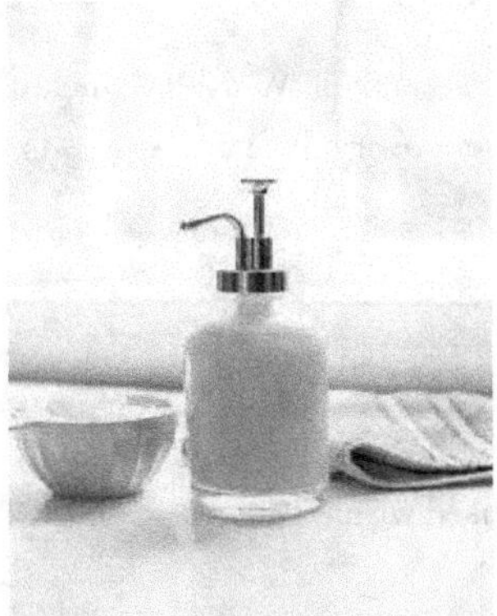

Ingredients:

- ¼ cup cocoa butter, melted
- ¼ cup coconut oil
- 3 tablespoons vegetable glycerin
- 1 tablespoon xanthan gum
- 1 cup grated castile soap
- 1 cup warm, distilled water
- 30 drops lavender essential oil
- Container (clean and sterile)
- Immersion Blender (or whisk)

Instructions:

1. In a bowl, combine the melted cocoa butter, coconut oil, vegetable glycerin, and xanthan gum. Stir gently and let the mixture sit for 5 minutes.

2. Using an immersion blender (or a whisk if you do not have one), blend the mixture until it begins to emulsify.

3. Add the castile soap, warm water, and lavender essential oil. Whisk or quickly blend the ingredients for just a couple of seconds. Do not over mix and create suds.

4. Let the mixture settle for 1-2 minutes.

5. Pour the gel into an appropriate container, and store it in a cool, dry place.

6. For best results, make small batches that will be used within 14 days.

To Use:

1. Shake the container gently before use.

2. Apply the cleanser to a sponge or washcloth and cleanse the body.

3. Rinse with comfortably warm water and gently pat dry when finished.

Rosemary and Tea Tree Aloe Shower Gel

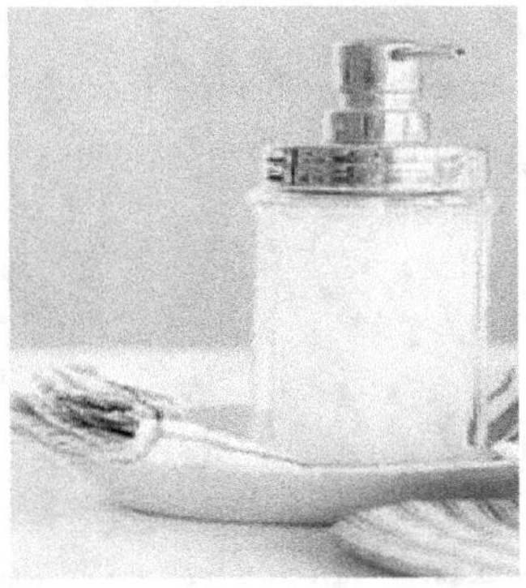

Ingredients:

- ¼ cup shea butter, melte
- cup apricot oil
- aloe vera gel
- vegetable glycerin
- xanthan gum
- distilled water
- rosemary essential oil
- tea tree essential oil
- Container (clean and sterile)
- Immersion blender (or a whisk)

Instructions:

1. In a bowl, combine the melted shea butter, apricot oil, aloe vera gel, vegetable glycerin, and xanthan gum. Stir gently and let the mixture sit for 5 minutes.

2. Using an immersion blender (or a whisk if you do not have one), blend the mixture until it begins to emulsify.

3. Add the castile soap, warm water, rosemary essential oil and tea tree essential oil. Whisk or quickly blend the ingredients for just a couple of seconds. Do not over mix and create suds.

4. Let the mixture settle for 1-2 minutes.

5. Pour the gel into an appropriate container, and store it in a cool, dry place.

6. For best results, make small batches that will be used within 14 days.

To Use:

1. Shake the container gently before use.

2. Apply the cleanser to a sponge or washcloth and cleanse the body.

3. Rinse with comfortably warm water and gently pat dry when finished.

Green Tea and Lemon Essence Shower Gel

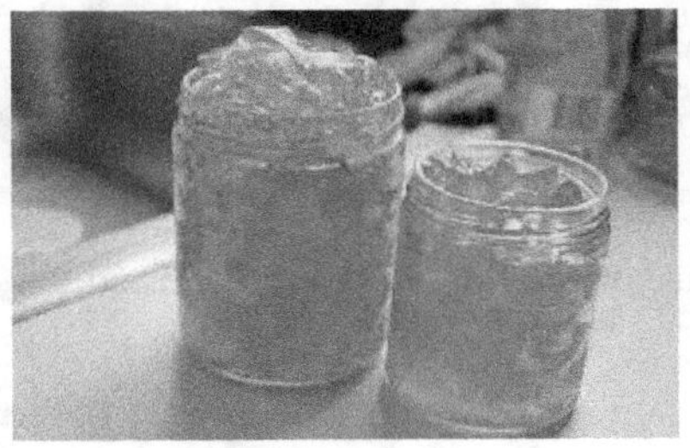

Ingredients:

- 1 cup warm, distilled water
- 2 organic green tea teabags
- ¼ cup shea butter, melted
- ¼ cup sweet almond oil
- 1 tablespoon vitamin E oil
- 1 tablespoon witch hazel
- 3 tablespoons vegetable glycerin
- 1 tablespoon xanthan gum
- 1 cup grated castile soap
- 15 drops lemon essential oil
- 5 drops rosemary essential oil (as a preservative) Container (clean and sterile)
- Immersion blender (or a whisk)

Instructions:

1. Begin by heating the distilled water until it is steamy, and then steeping the tea bags until the temperature of the water cools to warm and not hot.

2. Remove the tea bags and strain any tea leaves from the brewed tea.

3. In a bowl, combine the melted shea butter, sweet almond oil oil, vitamin E oil, witch hazel, vegetable glycerin, and xanthan gum. Stir gently and let the mixture sit for 5 minutes.

4. Using an immersion blender (or a whisk if you do not have one), blend the mixture until it begins to emulsify.

5. Add the castile soap, brewed tea, lemon essential oil and rosemary essential oil. Whisk or quickly blend the ingredients for just a couple of seconds. Do not over mix and create suds.

6. Let the mixture settle for 1-2 minutes.

7. Pour the gel into an appropriate container, and store it in a cool, dry place.

8. For best results, make small batches that will be used within 14 days.

To Use:

1. Shake the container gently before use.

2. Apply the cleanser to a sponge or washcloth and cleanse the body.

3. Rinse with comfortably warm water and gently pat dry when finished.

Vanilla Milk and Honey Shower Gel

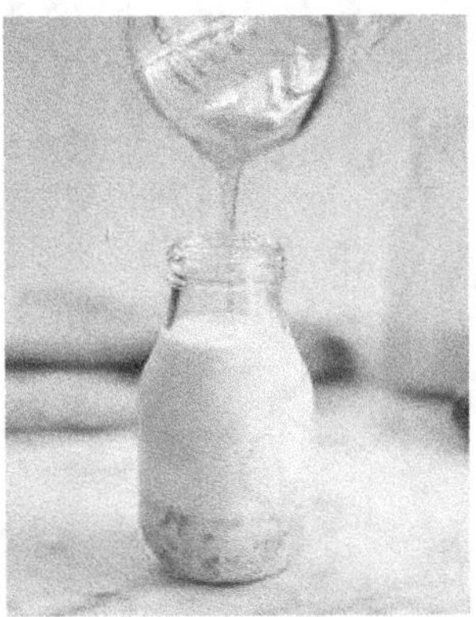

Ingredients:

- 1 cup liquid castile soap
- 1 cup coconut oil
- 1 cup local honey
- ¼ cups powdered coconut milk
- 15 drops vanilla absolute
- 5 drops rosemary essential oil (as a preservative) Container (clean and sterile)
- Immersion blender (or a whisk)

Instructions:

1. In a bowl, combine the liquid castile soap, coconut oil, honey, powdered coconut milk, vanilla absolute, and rosemary essential oil.

2. Let the mixture settle for 1-2 minutes.

3. Using an immersion blender (or a whisk if you do not have one), blend the mixture just long enough for it to emulsify. Try to avoid mixing it to the point that suds appear.

4. Pour the gel into an appropriate container, and store it in a cool, dry place.

5. For best results, make small batches that will be used within 14 days.

To Use:

1. Shake the container gently before use.

2. Apply the cleanser to a sponge or washcloth and cleanse the body.

3. Rinse with comfortably warm water and gently pat dry when finished.

Bees Knees Citrus Honey Wash

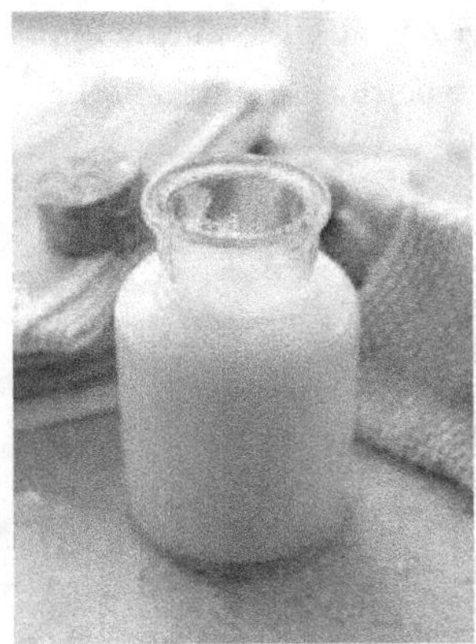

Ingredients:

- 1 cup liquid castile soap
- ¼ cup local honey
- 1 tablespoon vegetable glycerin
- 1 tablespoon vitamin E oil
- 1 tablespoon apricot kernel oil
- 10 drops sweet orange essential oil
- 5 drops grapefruit essential oil
- 5 drops lime essential oil
- 5 drops vanilla absolute
- Container (clean and sterile)
- Immersion blender (or a whisk)

Instructions:

1. In a bowl, combine the castile soap, local honey, vegetable glycerin, vitamin E oil, apricot kernel oil, sweet orange essential oil, grapefruit essential oil, lime essential oil, and vanilla absolute.

2. Let the mixture sit for 1-2 minutes.

3. Using an immersion blender (or a whisk if you do not have one), quickly blend the mixture just until it begins to emulsify. Try to avoid creating suds.

4. Pour the gel into an appropriate container, and store it in a cool, dry place.

5. For best results, make small batches that will be used within 14 days.

To Use:

1. Shake the container gently before use.

2. Apply the cleanser to a sponge or washcloth and cleanse the body.

3. Rinse with

Chapter 3. Conditioning Shampoos

Watermelon Delight Liquid Soap

This soap smells just like a fresh in half. It smells so yummy you will want to eat watermelon after you use it.

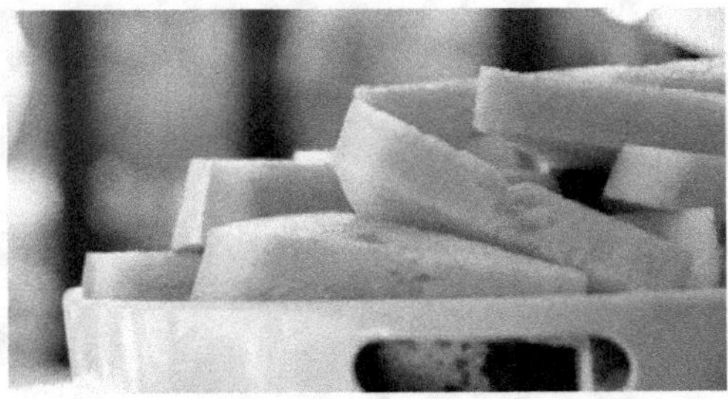

Makes: 8 oz. jar
Prep: 7 minutes

Ingredients:

- sweet almond oil
- vitamin E oil
- distilled water
- unscented castile soap
- watermelon fragrance oil

Instructions:

1. In an 8-ounce jar.

2. Add the distilled water first.

3. Then add the castile soap.

4. Lastly, add all the oils.

5. Shake before using.

Very Peary Liquid Soap

The smell of this fresh pear soap is enticing. It will make you smell so sweet that everybody will want to be around you.

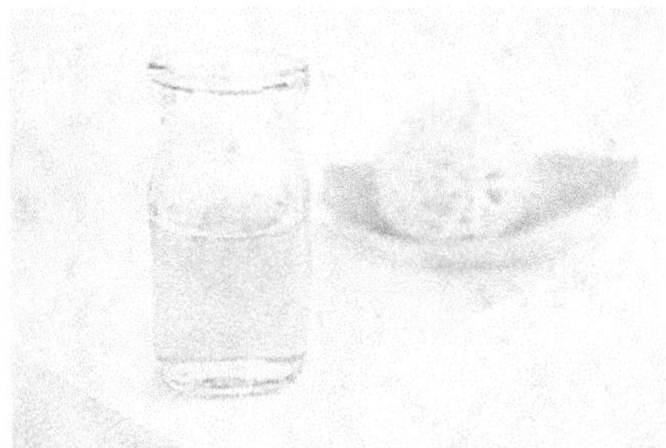

Makes: 16 ounces
Prep: 5 minutes

Ingredients:

- 1 cup peppermint castile soap
- 1 cup organic vegetable glycerin
- 2 tablespoons of grapeseed oil
- 20 drops of pear fragrance oil
- ½ teaspoon of vanilla extract

Instructions:

1. In a large bowl mix the castile soap and the glycerin.

2. Next add all the oils.

3. Pour in a container.

4. Shake before each use.

5. Enjoy!

Breathe Liquid Soap

Breathe is a clean air smelling soap. With the hint of spearmint to smell super refreshed and ready to go.

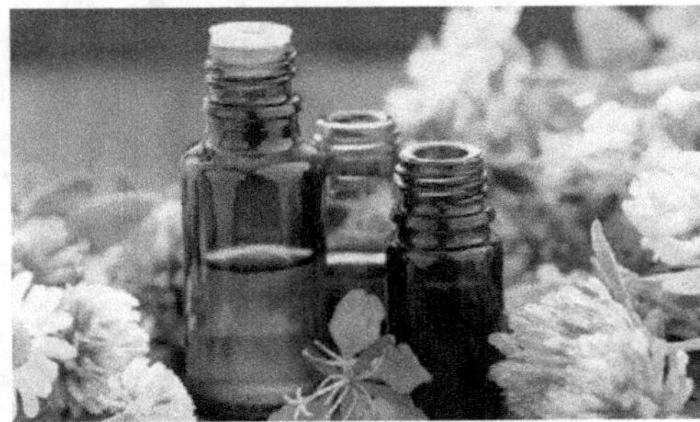

Makes: 8 oz. jar
Prep: 7 minutes

Ingredients:

- 1 tablespoon of avocado oil
- 1 tablespoon of vitamin E oil
- ½ cup of distilled water
- ½ cup unscented castile soap
- 2 drops eucalyptus essential oil
- 1 drop of spearmint essential oil
- 1 drop lemon essential oil

Instructions:

1. In an 8-ounce jar.

2. Add the distilled water first.

3. Then add the castile soap.

4. Lastly, add all the oils.

5. Shake before using.

Pumpkin Roll Liquid Soap

This soap smells like a fall day of baking pumpkin anything in the kitchen. It might even remind you of being at your grandmas baking with her when you were younger.

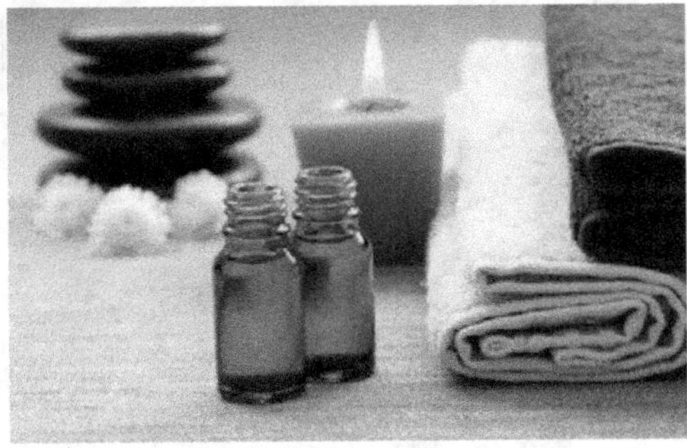

Makes: 9-pint sized jars
Prep: 20 minutes

Ingredients:

- 8 1 oz. bars of grated soap
- 2 tablespoons of vegetable glycerin
- 1 gallon of distilled water
- 2 drops of cinnamon essential oil
- 1 drop of ginger root essential oil
- 1 drop of vanilla essential oil
- 1 drop of pecan fragrance oil

Instructions:

1. Pour water into a large pot and warm on the stove.

2. Once its heated pour in the grated soap.

3. Mix until the soap is dissolved.

4. Pour in the glycerin.

5. Add in the essential oils.

6. Transfer to a large container.

7. Let it sit overnight.

8. Whisk the next morning.

9. Start using.

Strawberry Vanilla Liquid Soap

This liquid soap has a very pleasing scent. It is just like walking through a strawberry field with a hint of vanilla.

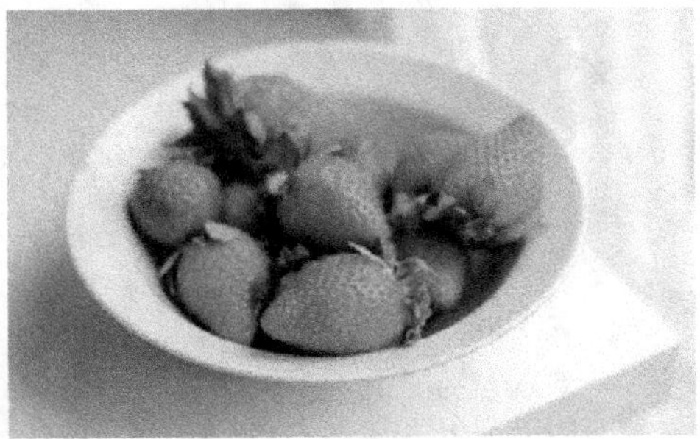

Makes: 8 oz. jar
Prep: 7 minutes

Ingredients:

- 1 tablespoon of castor oil
- 1 tablespoon of vitamin E oil
- ½ cup of distilled water
- ½ cup unscented castile soap
- 6 drops of strawberry fragrance oil
- 2 drops of vanilla essential oil

Instructions:

1. In an 8-ounce jar.

2. Add the distilled water first.

3. Then add the castile soap.

4. Lastly, add all the oils.

5. Shake before using.

Peppermint Dreams Liquid Soap

This smells just like a peppermint patty. Peppermint is great for helping you wake up, which is complemented with just a hint of chocolate aroma Perfect for any chocolate lover out there.

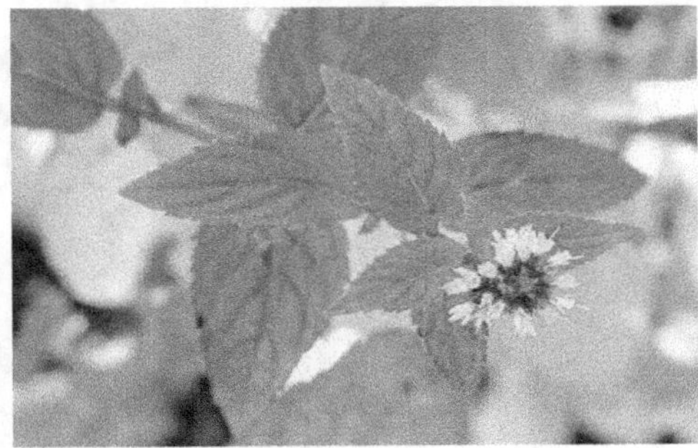

Makes: 9-pint sized jars
Prep: 20 minutes

Ingredients:

- 8 1 oz. bars of grated soap
- 2 tablespoons of vegetable glycerin
- 1 gallon of distilled water
- 3 drops of peppermint essential oil
- 1 drop of chocolate fragrance oil
- 1 drop of vanilla essential oil

Instructions:

1. Pour water into a large pot and warm on the stove.

2. Once its heated pour in the grated soap.

3. Mix until the soap is dissolved.

4. Pour in the glycerin.

5. Add in the essential oils.

6. Transfer to a large container.

7. Let it sit overnight.

8. Whisk the next morning.

9. Start using.

Chapter 4. Soaps for Children

Scooby Doo Soap

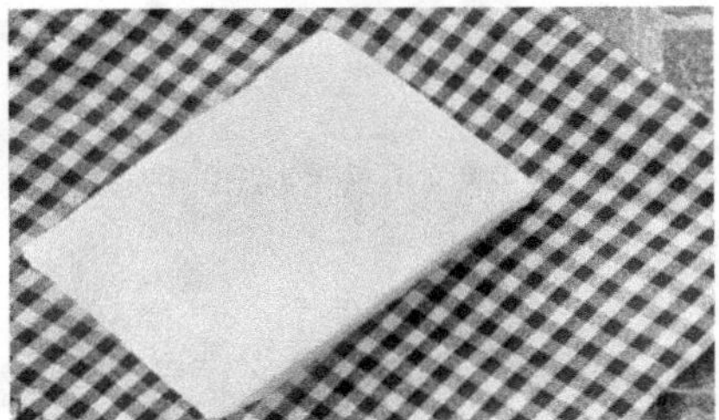

Get your kids looking and smelling clean with this organic homemade soap.

Ingredients

- 12 oz. of coconut oil
- 9.6 oz. of hemp seed oil
- 2.4 oz. of olive oil
- 14.4 oz. of palm oil
- 9.6 oz. of lye
- 15.84 oz. of water
- 0.50 oz. of rosewood essential oil
- 0.50 oz. of chamomile essential oil
- 0.50 oz. of mandarin essential oil

Instructions:

1. Pour all of the oils into a large crock pot and combine with a handheld mixer.

2. In a separate pan combine the water and the lye over high heat and stir until the lye dissolves.

3. Pour the lye mixture into the crockpot and combine with the handheld mixer until you start to see trails. This is referred to as tracing.

4. Put a lid onto the crock pot and allow the Ingredients to cook for 25 minutes.

5. Remove the lid, continue to stir and then cover and cook for another 10 minutes.

6. Test the Ingredients with a litmus strip, if it is still acidic continue to cook for a further 10 minutes and test again.

7. Once the Ingredients are no longer acidic they are ready to pour into the mold to finish curing.

8. Leave it to set overnight.

To Use

Wet the soap and rub it onto a body cloth until it lavers up.

Mickey Mouse Soap

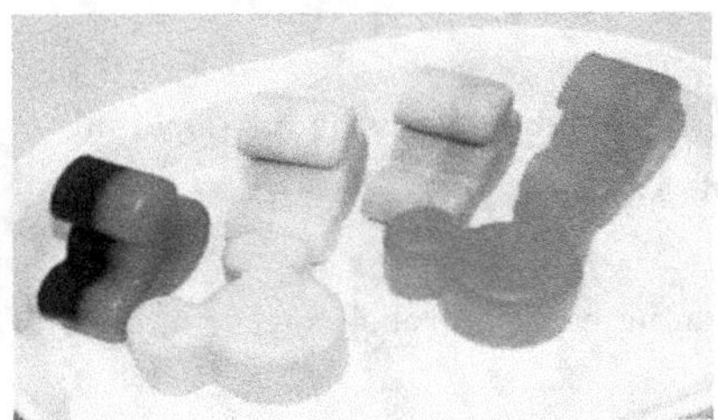

What better way to convince your kids to take a bath than with a soap named after their favorite cartoon character.

Ingredients

- 12 oz. of coconut oil
- 9.6 oz. of hemp seed oil
- 2.4 oz. of olive oil
- 14.4 oz. of palm oil
- 9.6 oz. of olive oil
- 7.13 oz. of lye oil
- 15.84 oz. of water
- 0.50 oz. of rosewood essential oil
- 0.50 oz. of chamomile essential oil
- 0.50 oz. of mandarin essential oil

Instructions:

1. Pour all of the oils into a large crock pot and combine with a handheld mixer.

2. In a separate pan combine the water and the lye over high heat and stir until the lye dissolves.

3. Pour the lye mixture into the crockpot and combine with the handheld mixer until you start to see trails. This is referred to as tracing.

4. Put a lid onto the crock pot and allow the Ingredients to cook for 25 minutes.

5. Remove the lid, continue to stir and then cover and cook for another 10 minutes.

6. Test the Ingredients with a litmus strip, if it is still acidic continue to cook for a further 10 minutes and test again.

7. Once the Ingredients are no longer acidic they are ready to pour into the mold to finish curing.

8. Leave it to set overnight.

To Use

Wet the soap and rub it onto a body cloth until it lavers up.

Smurfs Soap for Dry Oily Skin

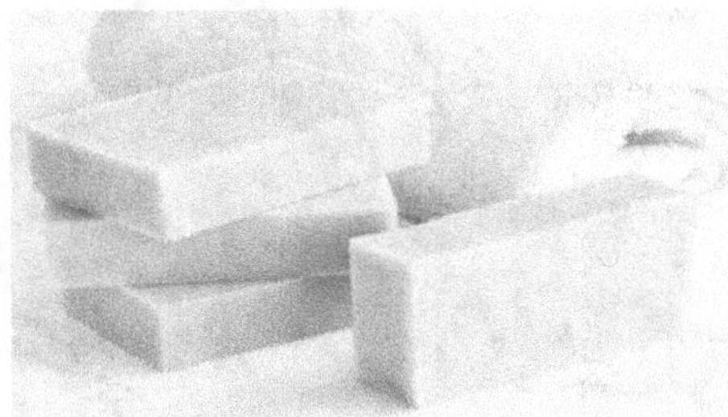

Kids can have skin problems too, but this homemade soap will soon get rid of it.

Ingredients

- 12 oz. of coconut oil
- 26.40 oz. of olive oil
- 9.6 oz. of palm oil
- 7.06 oz. of lye
- 15.84 oz. of water
- 0.75 oz. of frankincense essential oil
- 0.75 oz. of mandarin essential oil

Instructions:

1. Pour all of the oils into a large crock pot and combine with a handheld mixer.

2. In a separate pan combine the water and the lye over high heat and stir until the lye dissolves.

3. Pour the lye mixture into the crockpot and combine with the handheld mixer until you start to see trails. This is referred to as tracing.

4. Put a lid onto the crock pot and allow the Ingredients to cook for 25 minutes.

5. Remove the lid, continue to stir and then cover and cook for another 10 minutes.

6. Test the Ingredients with a litmus strip, if it is still acidic continue to cook for a further 10 minutes and test again.

7. Once the Ingredients are no longer acidic they are ready to pour into the mold to finish curing.

8. Leave it to set overnight.

To Use

Wet the soap and rub it onto a face cloth until it lavers up and wash the face as normal.

Daffy Duck Soap for Dry Skin

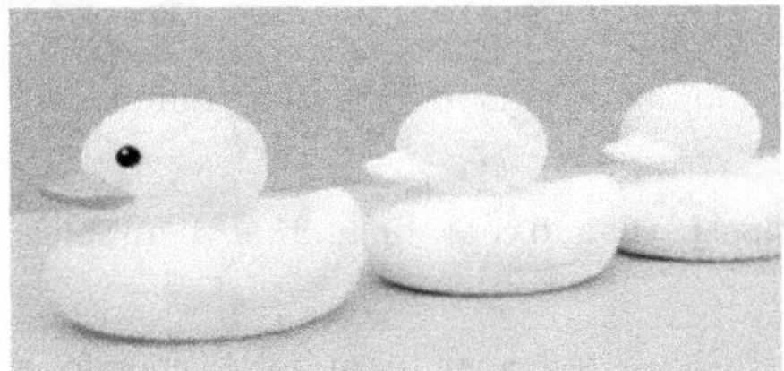

Dry skin in children is pretty common; the good news is you can get rid of it pretty quickly with this homemade chemical free soap.

Ingredients

- 12 oz. of coconut oil
- 26.40 oz. of olive oil
- 9.6 oz. of palm oil
- 7.06 oz. of lye
- 15.84 oz. of water
- 0.75 oz. of frankincense essential oil
- 0.75 oz. of mandarin essential oil

Instructions:

1. Pour all of the oils into a large crock pot and combine with a handheld mixer.

2. In a separate pan combine the water and the lye over high heat and stir until the lye dissolves.

3. Pour the lye mixture into the crockpot and combine with the handheld mixer until you start to see trails. This is referred to as tracing.

4. Put a lid onto the crock pot and allow the Ingredients to cook for 25 minutes.

5. Remove the lid, continue to stir and then cover and cook for another 10 minutes.

6. Test the Ingredients with a litmus strip, if it is still acidic continue to cook for a further 10 minutes and test again.

7. Once the Ingredients are no longer acidic they are ready to pour into the mold to finish curing.

8. Leave it to set overnight.

To Use

Wet the soap and rub it onto a body cloth until it lavers up.

Conclusion

Thank you for downloading this book; it is my sincere hope that you will apply the acquired knowledge on liquid soap making productively.

You will soon make the best liquid soaps ever and you will impress everyone around you with your homemade liquid soaps!

Just trust us! Get your ingredients ready and enjoy every recipe on this useful liquid soap collection. Start your new experience!

Have fun!

www.ingramcontent.com/pod-product-compliance
Lightning Source LLC
Chambersburg PA
CBHW051841250726

48659CB00005B/1961